A DOOR OF HOPE

A Door of Hope

Jean Vanier

Compiled by Anne-Sophie Andreu and
edited by Michel Quoist
Translated by Teresa de Bertodano

Hodder & Stoughton
LONDON SYDNEY AUCKLAND

Photographs on pages 11 and 38 by Toby Glanville
Used by permission.

Copyright © Jean Vanier 1996

Originally published by
Les Editions de l'Atelier, Paris, France.
First published in Great Britain 1996

10 9 8 7 6 5 4 3 2 1

British Library Cataloguing in Publication Data
A record for this book is available from the British Library

ISBN 0 340 63060 4

Typeset by Hewer Text Composition Services, Edinburgh
Printed and bound in Great Britain by
Cox & Wyman, Reading, Berks

Hodder and Stoughton Ltd
A Division of Hodder Headline PLC
338 Euston Road
London NW1 3BH

CONTENTS

Translator's Note

Much of the material in this book has already appeared in English and is reproduced from published sources. It has not, however, been possible to trace an existing English translation in all cases although every effort has been made to do so.

Some of the English texts were originally published over twenty years ago and slight adjustment has been made where appropriate. In addition, the author has slightly revised certain texts for the English translation of this book.

The phrase 'people with mental handicaps' is used to describe the men and women at the heart of l'Arche and Faith and Light communities. It is acknowledged that other terminology is in use but varies from one English-speaking country to another, e.g. 'people with learning difficulties', 'people with intellectual disabilities'. The existing phrase is used in the absence of a universally acceptable and accessible designation.

In France there are no specialist mental handicap hospitals. For this reason the term 'psychiatric hospital' has been retained in the English translation.

Very grateful thanks are due to Dr Thérèse Vanier for her help and advice which have clarified the text and improved the English.

Teresa de Bertodano

INTRODUCTION

In 1964 Jean Vanier bought a small house in the French village of Trosly-Breuil and moved into it with Raphaël Simi and Philippe Seux, two men with mental handicaps. Jean called the house l'Arche – the Ark – and in taking this first step he never imagined that thirty years later there would be 103 such communities in 28 countries, nor that this tiny opening in the wall of pain would become a door of hope for many others.

In taking this first step, Jean was answering two calls which are in reality a single call. The first call is that of Jesus Christ to the rich young man: 'Come, sell all that you have and follow me.' The second call came from those whom Jean had met in psychiatric hospitals, rejected by a society which was frightened by what they ask of it. In starting l'Arche, Jean was in fact answering the call to a life of love, tenderness, joy, forgiveness and compassion.

In answering it, he was also accepting the reality of pain, both for himself and for those whom he welcomed into his home, recognising that this pain could also reveal the grace of God in a mysterious way.

In these pages, Jean Vanier speaks to us of what he knows to be true: the love of God and the love of men and women, the tenderness and compassion of the poor and humble and the joy of simply being together. He also tells us of the fragility and distress of those who are weak and rejected, and reminds us of the hardness of our

1

own wounded hearts. Jean Vanier writes and talks and travels the world, tirelessly announcing the Good News of the Kingdom of God, built on the 'stone rejected by the builders which has become the cornerstone'. It is not the teaching of twentieth-century society and while we know what Jean is saying and would even like to believe him, the sad reality is that we do not think that it is possible.

And yet the communities of l'Arche in all their fragility and weakness are living proof that Jean is telling us the truth. Whoever we are and wherever we live, we too can make the choice to welcome others rather than to reject them, to live with one another in a spirit of acceptance and communion rather than in an atmosphere of competition where those who are 'different' and not so clever are automatically excluded. Jean is inviting us to join him in this way of life. He is telling us that we no longer have to be afraid or to defend ourselves against one another and – more significantly – that we do not have to defend ourselves against what is inside our own hearts. He is telling us that we can choose life rather than death.

This was the choice that Jean made and it led him to begin l'Arche.

A Door of Hope gives us a brief outline of his life followed by extracts from his writings and conferences, illustrated by photographs of l'Arche in different countries. The book is based on the text of Micah 6:8.

> You have already been told what is right
> and what the Lord requires of you:
> only this:
> act justly,
> love tenderly,
> walk humbly with your God.

Introduction

L'Arche is primarily a work of justice and wants to respond in a spirit of welcome and deep commitment to the cry of pain in those who are excluded from our society. But l'Arche is also aware that justice without love can never be sufficient and that it is necessary to risk loving and committing one's life in compassion and tenderness. L'Arche has discovered, just as we too can discover if we are willing to take the same road, that God is walking with each of us and that it is the poor who reveal the true face of God, our gentle shepherd.

A *Door of Hope* brings together three different sorts of text: those which give an indication of the philosophy behind l'Arche and are perhaps more 'theoretical', contemplative passages describing the spirituality of l'Arche, and descriptive writings which are illustrated with photographs and describe daily life within l'Arche communities. More than anything else this is what l'Arche is about: people who are at home in themselves, as witnessed in their faces and in their looks and gestures of relationship. In this being at home the most humble and simple daily life (enlightened from within) reveals its true identity – that is, the place of the infinitely fragile presence of God.

Anne-Sophie Andreu

FOLLOWING JESUS

Jean Vanier, A Portrait

Following Jesus

I live with people who cannot speak, who are rejected, seen as 'mad' and all too often kept away from the Good News of Jesus.

Nothing in my early life prepared me for this. My father was a diplomat and I was born in Switzerland in 1928 while he was serving there as military adviser to the Canadian delegation to the League of Nations. Most of my early childhood was spent in England and France until 1940 when France fell and we left Europe for Canada.

At the age of thirteen I wanted to join the Royal Navy. When I asked my father's permission, he replied, 'If you feel that this is what you really want to do, then go, I trust you.' I have always been grateful to my parents for taking me seriously and for the trust they placed in me. Their confidence enabled me to trust myself and also gave me a sense of responsibility and an awareness that my own intuition was trustworthy.

I returned to England and spent the next three years at the Naval College in Dartmouth followed by four years serving as a naval officer aboard different ships.

The war affected me profoundly. Shortly after the liberation of Paris I found myself at a railway station there, welcoming survivors from Buchenwald, Dachau, Belsen and Auschwitz. I shall never forget those men and women coming off the trains like skeletons, their faces tortured by fear, anguish and pain, still wearing their white-striped uniforms.

It seemed to me unbearable that human beings could torture others like this because of their hatred and their need to crush others. Horrible, too, that tens of thousands were killed in an instant when the atomic bombs exploded over Hiroshima and Nagasaki in 1945.

'Follow me'

In 1948 I transferred to the Canadian navy and later served in the aircraft carrier *Magnificent*. Although it was a way of life that I loved, I found myself increasingly drawn towards prayer, the Gospels and spiritual things in general. It was becoming apparent that Jesus wanted me to leave the navy to work for peace rather than for war. It took two years for the grace of God to deepen in me; in 1950 I resigned from the navy to follow Jesus. Everything else flowed from that decision.

My first step was to go to a Christian community near Paris to study philosophy and do some manual work. I later spent twelve months living as a guest in a Trappist monastery, followed by two years at Fatima in Portugal, and then, on receiving my doctorate, I went back to Toronto to teach philosophy at the university.

In 1963, on a visit to France, I went to see Père Thomas Philippe who had helped me and guided me in 1950 when I left the navy. He was serving as chaplain to the Val Fleuri, a house for thirty men with mental handicaps. Père Thomas introduced me to a world of suffering of which I had been completely unaware. I was shocked by the pain of these men and the cry that came from them – 'Do you love me?', 'Why have I been abandoned?', 'Why can't I be like my married brothers and sisters who have their own homes?' They were yearning, crying out for love. This primal cry exists within each of us, however much we try to cover it over with ideas and things to 'do'.

That first meeting touched me deeply. I began to visit psychiatric hospitals and to discover the pain of

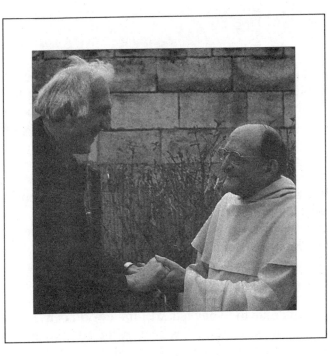

Jean and Père Thomas Philippe

people who have mental handicaps. I saw that they were amongst the most oppressed people of our world. They had no voice in our society. People feared them, turned away from them, wanted to get rid of them.

The beginning

Père Thomas encouraged me to buy a small house near Compiègne in the village of Trosly–Breuil. I invited two men with mental handicaps whom I had met in a psychiatric hospital to come and live with me, Raphaël Simi and Philippe Seux – and that was the beginning of l'Arche.

I knew this was an irreversible act, that there was no turning back. I wanted to live with them, to give them a family, a community, a place to belong. And this could only happen if we all lived together, with Raphaël and Philippe at the heart of things.

At first I thought that I would be able to help them to 'do' things, but I soon found that we were helping each other; Raphaël and Philippe were teaching me about becoming human. They led me into a world of friendship and communion which was healing me and bringing me new life. Obviously I knew how to 'do' plenty of things – I could teach and organise and all the rest – but that was not what they wanted most of all. They needed me to be with them, to love them and to establish relationship with them.

And then . . .

Friends soon came to help. Little by little, we welcomed other men; the community grew and we began to open houses for women. There were soon several houses in

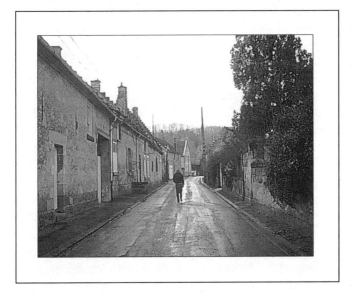

The first l'Arche house is in Trosly-Breuil, France

Trosly and the neighbouring villages, and in 1970 we began communities in other parts of France and also in Canada and India.

The Bangalore foundation was important for me as it introduced me to the Third World in all its grandeur and suffering. Visits to India brought a new awareness of the problems of our world and, in particular, of the gravity of the times in which we live.

Gandhi is often misunderstood in the West but I found him to be one of the great prophets of today. I learnt that his great love for the 'untouchables' was deeply rooted in his life of prayer and I discovered his 'littleness' before the God of Love, his thirst for justice and his desire for unity between peoples divided by religion. Mahatma Gandhi, who so loved the Beatitudes, casts new light on the teaching of Jesus.

The ecumenical aspect of l'Arche has been extremely important and its significance became apparent through our foundations in countries where the principal Christian denomination was other than Roman Catholic. The fact that communities were also coming to birth in countries without any significant Christian tradition was equally important in revealing the interfaith aspect of l'Arche.

It is as if the unifying factor for those of any religion or of none is the willingness to work for people who are 'poor' in the eyes of the world while recognising their particular contribution. My personal belief is that in this way a man or woman with a mental handicap can be a force for Christian unity. Even if we are not all able to drink from a single Eucharistic cup we can share in the same cup of suffering and we can eat together at the same table.

I believe that in a small way our communities are the sign of an existing unity as well as an indication of the way in which greater unity can be achieved. There are now 103 of them in 28 countries, including those of the Eastern Bloc, such as Hungary and Poland. Most of the communities consist of several houses where people with mental handicaps and their assistants live as a family.

Needs vary according to country. In some places we have workshops, while in Burkina Faso, West Africa, we have a school. Our principal aim is to be part of the wider community, sharing in the activities of the neighbourhood; the last thing we want is the sort of self-sufficiency which would turn us into a ghetto.

Faith and Light

Faith and Light was born in 1971 following a pilgrimage to Lourdes organised by Marie-Hélène Mathieu and myself, in response to a request from parents of people with a mental handicap. There are now some 1250 Faith and Light communities in 65 countries.

While the basic vision is similar to that of l'Arche, members of Faith and Light communities do not live under the same roof. Instead they gather together regularly: people with mental handicaps, their parents and friends meeting as a group in which those who are least able from a human point of view are fully recognised and accepted. Faith and Light communities are oases of peace and love to which people with mental handicaps can bring their own contribution and especially their ability to love other people as they are.

Blessed are the poor

Through living with Raphaël and Philippe and others like them, I gradually started to see the world through new eyes. Thanks to them, I became aware that the

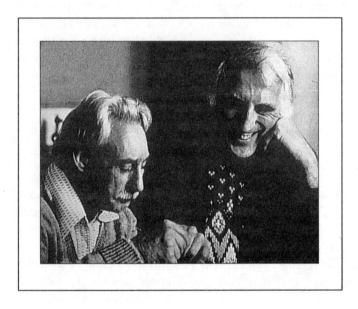

Jean and Raphaël at Trosly-Breuil

teaching of the Gospels is totally at odds with our twentieth-century society in which any tendency towards compassion or togetherness is looked down upon while ambition, aggression and competition are lauded, alongside the search for riches and power.

Living as I do with people who have mental handicaps, I am very much aware of their inner beauty and tenderness of heart, while at the same time recognising their incapacities and the extent of their suffering. Thus I have come to understand the close link described in the Gospels between God in his infinite greatness and the person who counts for nothing by human reckoning. The truth is that the greater the poverty of an individual, the more powerfully God seems to be present. Jesus reveals his special love for those who are cast aside by the world. And Saint Paul reiterates the teaching. 'God has chosen what is foolish by human reckoning to confound the wise, he has chosen what is weak by human reckoning to confound the strong, those who by human reckoning are common and contemptible, those who count for nothing.' (1 Cor. 1: 27–8).

And Jesus goes still further. He himself became poor and was cast aside and he reveals that he is now one with the poor – and we find this to be so in our communities. Jesus is very specially present in those who are least by our human standards. L'Arche is founded on the certain knowledge that the poor have a special and privileged place in the Kingdom of God and that we 'assistants' are called to walk with them. It is a journey which includes experiences of togetherness, peace, celebration and forgiveness, just as it involves the discovery and acceptance of our own weakness and poverty – everything that we try to conceal behind our capabilities and our capacity to 'get things done'. Even our so-called generosity can be a way of escaping from aspects of ourselves that we do not want to face.

A Door of Hope

Men and women with mental handicaps are frequently ignored and cast aside because their existence obliges us to face our own limitations, inner darkness and spiritual poverty. And yet, in rejecting these people, we are in fact running away from our true selves and refusing to allow the man or woman with a mental handicap to reveal to us that we are loved, exactly as we are.

Like the Gospels, l'Arche is a paradox. In it we discover something unexpected and shocking. The man or woman with a mental handicap, perceived by society as a problem, useless, a burden, we see as a source of life, drawing us towards truth, towards Jesus and the Gospel.

For me, to follow Jesus is to be with those who have been cast aside and to meet him in and with them.

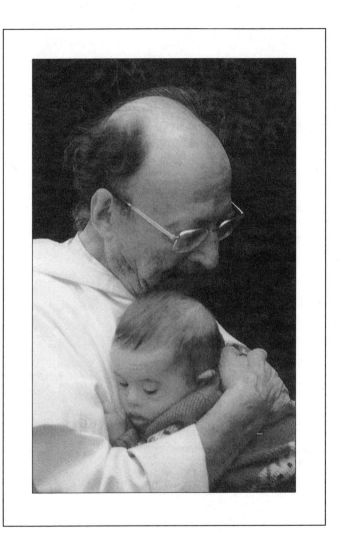

Père Thomas embraces a young child

ACT JUSTLY

People in misery are crushèd
    encircled
    without hope of rising by themselves

surrounded and knotted with obstacles and difficulties
    no desire
    no hope
    no motivation
    no will to live
    closed off

people in misery are still there
    waiting . . . waiting . . .
    waiting for what?
    lying in their prison
    lying in their dung . . .
    waiting yet not waiting
    for they have lost hope

we only wait
    when there is hope
where there is no hope
    we lie dying
    not living
    sad unto death

yet they wait
    waiting . . . yet not waiting . . .

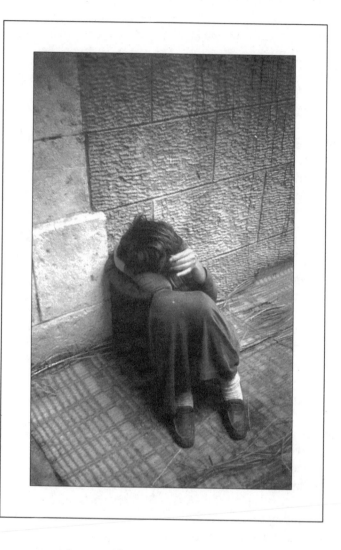

A young girl in an institution in Jerusalem

When I see Evelyn banging her head against the floor, when I hear Robert in the middle of the night begging someone to cut off his genitals, when I see Luke aimlessly running round and round, when I see the closed, tense face of George, I know in each there is a profound agony and an unbearable interior restlessness.

A baby who has a mental handicap, sensing that it is not wanted, will harden its heart and body and, to protect itself, will withdraw from reality. There is thus a sort of inner death: life no longer evolves. Agitation prevents development. Certain aspects of the psychic being become blocked. The brain, language and even physical development are all affected. Thus begins the fragmentation of the being.

I remember John Mark seated next to me in the chapel, whispering over and over: 'I have the devil in me. I have evil in me.' The story of John Mark is a story of rejection. Born in a psychiatric hospital, abandoned by his mother, he was adopted, but this did not work out. He then went from one foster family to another. After a time, he was placed in a small institution and then sent to a psychiatric hospital because he had shown signs of violence. At the age of twenty-seven, he came to l'Arche. Never in his life had he had a lasting and unique relationship with an adult. Moved from one place to another, he had never heard anyone say to him, 'You are my beloved son and you are my joy. Between us is an indestructible bond. No matter what you do, you will always be my child.' John Mark was without any roots.

The great question in each of us is: 'Am I of value? Is there someone who believes in me sufficiently to be concerned about me and to live a covenant relationship with me?' This is a cry for bonds of friendship and recognition which are experienced in different ways.

There is the cry to be loved by a father and mother who know how to hold one in one's weakness. It is a cry which springs from the fragility of the infant or the insecurity of the adolescent. It is the cry of the adult with a mental handicap who needs tenderness, welcome, kindness, compassion, personal nourishment, support and encouragement. It is a cry which says: 'I need you. Your love gives me life and roots.' It is also the cry of every human person, because each of us carries our fragilities and our difficulties. Each of us cries out to be loved by someone who will support us. It is also the cry which turns us to God.

Secondly, there is the cry for a friend, an equal, a brother or a sister. One is no longer a little child who is loved but a person able to love and make another happy in community life. This desire for friendship may become a search for the unique friend in love and marriage.

Finally, there is the call to be a friend to the weakest and to serve.

People with low self-esteem are sometimes described as 'marginal' but it is a word which can be applied to all of us. We all suffer from low self-esteem and do not really know who we are.

There are so many people living on the edge of despair, in the sort of misery that makes it impossible for them to be happy or creative. We are all damaged by sin and by our own moral or spiritual poverty – and I am not talking about poverty in the sense of 'blessed are the poor', but rather of the misery and despair that come from our weakness and infidelity and our inability to trust in the forgiveness of God.

We are all called by God – called to love – but we are broken and we do not know who we really are.

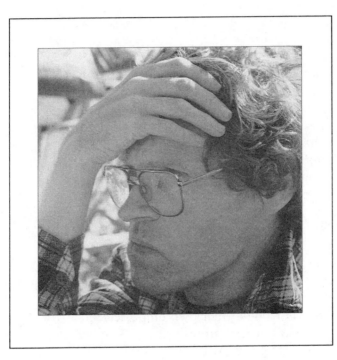

George from l'Arche Bognor Regis

The poor can be the economically poor,
who are hungry, homeless and out of work,
or the rejected ones –
those put aside because of their infirmities and
    handicaps,
their apparent uselessness.
They are longing to be accepted and loved,
longing for meaning and a healing relationship.

The poor are those caught up in sin,
yet craving also to be liberated from it.
The poor are also any of us
who are sad and alone, feeling guilty and unloved.

The poor know their own emptiness.
They do not hide from it.
They long for a saviour
who will heal their hearts
and bring them peace.

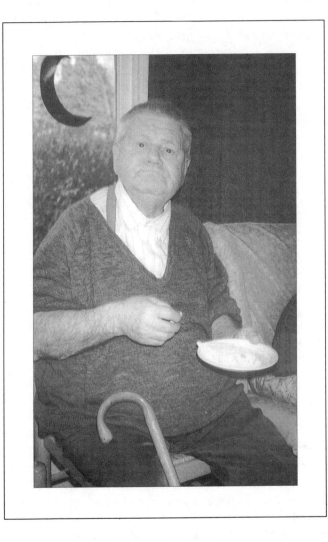

Ian from l'Arche Inverness

Do you really think, looking clearly at the facts, that our society can continue as it is now without committing collective suicide? Do you not realise that the grave injustices in the slums of South America, in the large cities of Europe and Asia, the injustices committed against black people in the United States and in Africa, the injustices throughout the world, are smouldering fires that may burst into flames in the near future? Do you not see that there are tremendous powers ready to unite the discontented and to stimulate the revolutionaries? Do you really believe that the world tensions: US–Russia, Russia–China, China–US, Eastern countries–Russia, Israel–Arabs, North and South Vietnam, etc., will not explode one day into a devastating fire and that we will not use the nuclear arms that science has put at our disposal? Do you really think that the inactivity of youth, their lack of ideal and the absence of motivation are not going to lead our society to despair? Do you not think that the terrible waste in the West in front of the penury and misery in other countries is going to arouse an aggressiveness that will overflow one day? Do you really think that we can continue with our compromising religions which make no real demands on our persons, with our system of middle-class, 'do-gooder' morality, with our luxurious neighbourhoods and large homes, and all of this next door to the slums and unending misery? Do you really think we can continue to propagate, through advertisements and propaganda, a morality of egotistic and materialistic pleasure when in reality, more than ever before, we need generosity and an ideal?

I am certain that this state of affairs cannot continue. Our society will be transformed through the fire of revolution or through the stagnant waters of decadence or through the fire and peace of true love. There is still time. But time is short.

To confront the seriousness of this crisis and in face of these grave injustices, a new race of men and women capable of great generosity is required.

For society to convert itself, or rather for men and women of today to turn away from materialistic egoism and from violence and revolution, the married couples of today must burn with new hearts and new spirits – hearts of flesh and spirits of fire as spoken of by the prophet Ezekiel (chapter 36).

There must be a more authentic receptivity and openness, a more radical poverty, greater hope and audacity, and a keener thirst for justice and truth. A new generation of men and women is needed who have complete confidence in the action of the Spirit of God and who will leave the security of the extended family of wealth and material welfare in order to live in the hands of God, so that they may spread the spirit of truth, peace and love in their own countries or in others where misery is more blatant.

A Door of Hope

Two prisons divided by a gulf,
the miserable person
I treat you as a stranger . . .
you were born and reared in squalor . . .
you are walled in, for you have no life
in front of you . . . no joys to look forward to . . .
no loving children . . . no esteem

I, with my clean clothes
my sensitive nose (I hate
bad smells) . . . my politeness . . .
a warm house . . . a world of security . . .
the light of reality does not penetrate
my cell, the reality
of human misery so widespread, so deep . . .

Two prisons divided by a gulf,
the miserable person . . . imprisoned . . .
and in the cell next door
the person of means comfortably installed . . .
and so the world goes on . . .
and the gulf gets wider . . .
who will be the bridge?

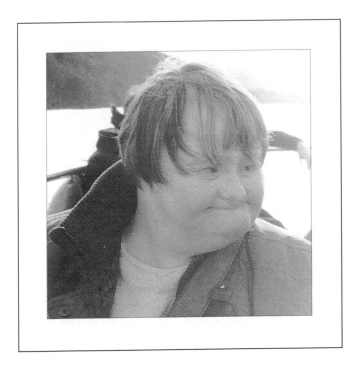

Jackie from l' Arche Inverness

Come, listen and learn.
Do not judge others and their ways;
instead respect them and love them.
Open your hearts to them.

If you come in this way,
open, listening humbly, without judging,
then gradually you will discover
that you are trusted.
Your heart will be touched.
You will begin to discover the secret of communion.

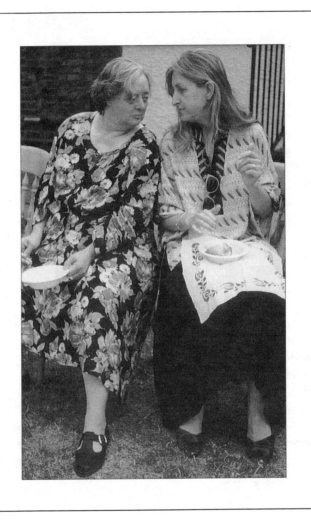

Doreen and Corinne at l'Arche Lambeth

Jesus came to announce peace. He has an extraordinary message for today: do not try to live according to the values of society, the values of riches, status and ambition. Just seek peace where you are and I will give you peace.

If you grow in peace through living the Gospel, simply and poorly, I will give you a hunger and thirst for justice which will be satisfied through gentleness. I will give you new strength, the power of the Spirit manifesting itself in mercy – blessed are the merciful. You will be compassionate towards those who are weakest and most despised – men and women coming out of prison or who are in psychiatric hospitals, those who are old or handicapped.

The important thing is to really meet other people. This is true mercy – to show compassion and bring true freedom through the way in which you listen – helping others to realise that they are precious and that you want them to be free because you love them and respect them. This is the way to build peace – to become a man or woman of peace.

How then to approach the child in misery?
not haughtily
but humbly
not judging
but loving

determined not to dominate
not even to give things
rather to give myself
my time, energy and heart

and to listen
believing that he or she is important
a child of God
in whom Jesus lives

approach with tenderness
gently
peacefully
graciously

We are called to open ourselves up to others. To really welcome others is a lengthy process. The importance of welcome cannot be over-emphasised. It lies at the heart of Christianity and is primarily a matter of becoming available to others. We cannot call ourselves followers of Jesus unless we are willing to open ourselves up to the real world and the joys and sorrows of those around us, accepting them as they are. It is hard to be welcoming because so often we close up upon ourselves and our problems; we are depressed or angry.

We are frightened of our human reality, frightened of all the pain in our world. There is so much misery, oppression, infidelity and hatred; so many wars; no wonder we tend to run away from reality and from people who ask of us what we cannot give.

And yet the 'barometer' of our physical and spiritual well-being is our willingness to welcome others. This is the sign of whether or not we are becoming truly human. Jesus calls us to love our humanity and to live as human beings, open one to another.

Look. Listen. Touch. Touch the wounded person, touch the hand, help him or her realise we are close. The Spirit leads us from stopping, to looking, to listening and then to touching, as we are drawn from our culture, our style of life, our pattern of thinking, the emphasis on particular forms and types of education. The Holy Spirit gradually breaks all these down, and allows us to listen to and look at people without fear.

This does not mean that tomorrow we start to throw our arms round people of other cultures. It doesn't work like that. To begin with, we should get down on our knees and ask the forgiveness of our wounded brothers and sisters, who today are still in hospitals, shut up because they were handicapped as children. Ask pardon of those who we have shut up behind prison bars because, in many ways, it is our attitudes that have pushed them there and keep them there. We send them back to prison because we do not welcome them when they come out.

We need to start by asking the forgiveness of God.

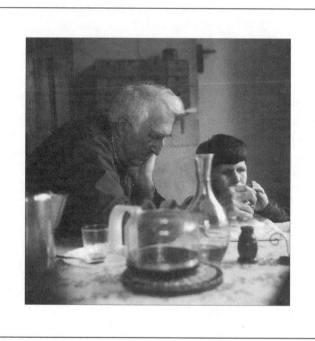

Jean and Loic at Trosly-Breuil

God entrusted to Joseph the only begotten Son, the Word. Joseph became responsible for the Word made flesh, Jesus, so that he might grow and accomplish his mission of love.

In L'Arche, God has entrusted to us many people. We are responsible for them. The paternity of Joseph is, of course, unique and special: the child was entrusted to him even before birth and this child is light born of light, true God born of true God. Each one of our people has a father according to the flesh; we can be but substitutes. Many have suffered rejection by their fathers and have a negative image of themselves. In them there is anger and depression: they are not all light. On the contrary, what is often most conspicuous is this world of darkness and desperation in them; the light often remains very hidden, concealed deep within their beings. Nevertheless, in their weakness and dependence, in their growing confidence, they resemble the little child entrusted to Joseph. We are responsible for them, for their well-being, for their development and growth. They have been entrusted to us just as l'Arche has been entrusted to us.

And if we do not fulfil our responsibility to them, they will not reach the plenitude of their being; they will not grow as they should. They will not be happy. They will not know freedom and peace of heart. They will not realise that they are loved by God and that they have a special place in the Church and in humanity. They will not be able to fulfil their mission. We are responsible for them, to liberate them through our love, to give them confidence in themselves through our confidence in them. We are responsible for confirming them and calling them forth to further growth, for nourishing their hope, their hearts and their bodies; for educating them and helping them to grow. Yes, it is a very great and marvellous responsibility that has been entrusted to each one of us.

It is Jesus' deepest desire that we be one as he and the Father are one.

In l'Arche we are called to live this unity in community. And so each one of us is called to die to selfishness, rivalry and to the need to prove oneself, in order to discover that difference is a treasure and not a threat. Our unity, and harmony in diversity, our respect for each other's gifts, our need for one another, to co-operate together, will be a source of much fecundity.

We are also called to live this unity in the larger family of l'Arche throughout the world. Our communities in India and Haiti are so different from the ones in England and Canada for example. We have different languages, races and religions. These differences are a treasure! Through them we can learn so much about ourselves, about others and about the ways of God.

Community is essentially a place where we learn to live in a way that meets our deepest needs. It is a coming together of people who want to show that it is possible to live, love, celebrate and work together for peace, justice and a better world. It is a sign that love is possible in a materialistic society where men and women ignore one another or even kill each other.

A community is like an orchestra playing a symphony. Every instrument by itself can play beautifully but it is even better when they all play together, each one making a unique and essential contribution.

It is the people who love, forgive and listen who build community. It is those who are sensitive, who serve others, and who nourish them and pray for them. And each of us, by the grace that has been given to us, exercises our gifts according to our own good and unique expression of love and tenderness. A community is only really a community when all its members realise how deeply they need the gifts of others, and try to make themselves more transparent and more faithful in the exercise of their own gift. So a community is built by every one of its members, each in their own way.

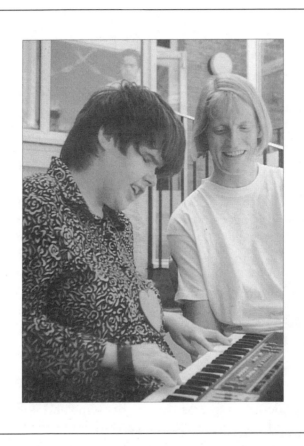

Sharon and Katherine at Lambeth

I love the image of the wounded bird held in the cupped hand. The hand is not too open, otherwise the bird might fall. It is not too closed for that might crush the bird. The hand is like a nest, it carries and gives support to the bird, communicating warmth and security to him so that when the right moment comes, he can regain strength and take off on his own. The father is like this cupped hand. He does not possess the child; he does not enclose him nor harm him, but he helps the child so that later he may take off on his own.

Our lives, our bodies, our communities, are called to be this cupped hand in order to receive and carry others. Not to possess, harm, judge or condemn them, but to carry them. To carry the weakest ones with their suffering, anger, depression, dreams, illusions, and lack of confidence as well as their light, hope and possibility for growth. We are called to carry them until they can take off on their own, and become more completely themselves, capable of choosing their new home.

LOVE TENDERLY

Adam loved Eve; Eve loved Adam.
They were one body, one love, one spirit.
Each one could give to the other,
each one could drink from the other.
Gentle communion,
gentle passion flowing one from another.
And this communion rose up as incense to God.
Their love, their gift of self to each other, their
    unity,
was a celebration, a thanksgiving, a praise.
God rejoiced to see their wholeness
and their joy in one another,
reflecting the glory of the divine.
And it was from the depth of their communion
    with God
and with each other
that they were destined to give birth to children,
and grow as a family,
develop the earth with all its potential
and consecrate it to God.

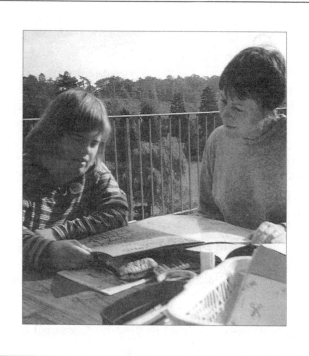

André and Carmel from Lambeth

Love is a much maligned word.

Real love is attentive, and concerned for the other person. It respects the person just as he or she is, acknowledging the bad but recognising the potential for growth, however well this may be concealed.

Love believes in the beloved, even when it seems crazy and hopeless, and rejoices in her inner beauty even when nobody else can see it. 'I don't care what they say. It doesn't always have to be like this. I believe in you and I know that you can do great things.'

Love rejoices in the presence of the other person and in the beauty of his or her heart even if it remains quite hidden.

Love creates deep and lasting bonds whatever the setbacks.

All too often we take an interest in someone only when we can 'do good' in order to 'feel good': in which case we are loving ourselves, trying to enhance our own self-image. It is only too easy to love people when it suits us so that we can feel 'useful' or even 'successful'. When they start to disturb us and make increasing demands we put up barriers in order to defend ourselves.

Real love is quite different. It is to forget ourselves sufficiently to allow our hearts to beat at the rhythm of another: it is to suffer alongside; it is compassion.

Innocente is part of our community in the Ivory Coast.

When we first met her she had been abandoned in the bush and left to die: a tiny little girl with a wasted body and no name. She was found by a passer-by who called her Innocente. Later she came to us.

Within a year Innocente began to discover that she was loved. She must be ten or eleven now and she is very beautiful. Her body quivers when you take her in your arms, and her eyes and her whole being say, 'I love you.'

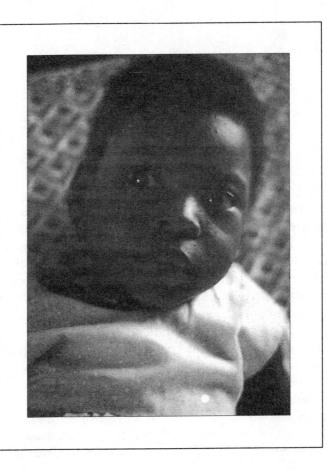

Innocente from the Ivory Coast

We are frightened of love because it implies risk. We cannot know how the other person might evolve. Perhaps I will be faithful but the other person will not be. Perhaps I will be the unfaithful one because I know I am weak. That is the risk of love.

We are also frightened of love because it is linked to procreation which is at the same time wonderful and very disturbing: wonderful in that the love between two people can bring forth new life, but disturbing because it introduces a dimension we would sometimes prefer to be without. It can be tempting to refuse the gift of new life and consider sexuality and procreation as separate entities. But it is logical that they should be linked, and remind lover and beloved of their responsibilities, not only to one another but to the universe.

There is something very beautiful in this physical consequence of love which reminds us deeply of what it means to be human, to be faithful. Love is the marriage between time and eternity: it roots us in present experience while opening us to the infinite. The beauty of love lies not only in the wonder of being together, but in deep fidelity, mutual affection and lasting commitment.

What is love, a myth or a reality? A true experience or an illusion? Is love a real goal or is it an escape? It is represented in multiple ways, on television, radio and in films. Is it an ephemeral attraction between man and woman which is expressed in the sex act? Is it a game, a pastime, an adventure, a desire to seduce or dominate? Or is it a human and even a divine reality, the summit of friendship implying a gift, an experience outside time and faithfulness within time?

Love is the highest and the most profound mystery of the universe, the source and end of all things, but it implies force of character, inner fidelity, intelligence, delicacy of heart and above all the capacity to listen, to accept and to place oneself at the disposition of the other. These attitudes are rare in our society, but rare things are often the most beautiful and the heart and mind must be opened out towards them.

It is the incomparable treasure of love and of union alone that can bring happiness.

A meeting
> is a strange and wonderful thing
> presence
> one person to another
> present
> one to another
> life flowing
> one to another

but
> we can be together
> and not meet
> we can live in the same house
> day after day
> sit at the same table
> kneel at the same pew
> read the same books
> but never meet

we can kiss
> gestures of love
> apparent tenderness
> but never meet

a meeting is a strange and wonderful thing
> presence one person to another
> present one to another
> life flowing one to another

And during all the time he hung there
    the woman was beside him.
A sign of hope, of trust, of love.
She stood firm,
this silent woman of compassion,
not crushed,
not fleeing from the pain.

It was fitting and right that she be full of grace,
overshadowed by the Spirit,
to love her child –
not clutching at him out of her own emptiness
with possessive love,
but loving him from the overflowing of her own
    fullness.

And in this grace she could know and hold him
in all his littleness and vulnerability.
She could respond to his cry for food
and for the food of love
to nourish his gentle heart
hungry for love, for communion and relationship.

So when he was led to the slaughter,
like a lamb, on Calvary,
she was not scandalised nor felt ashamed.
She loved him.

Let me tell you about Claudia who is blind, unable to relate and described as 'autistic'. She was abandoned by her family at a hospital in Tegucigalpa (Honduras). When she first came to our community she was frightened, disorientated, deeply disturbed and very insecure. She lived in a world of anguish and inner pain, cried out day and night, chewed her clothes and wiped excrement on the walls.

The community was very small with three excellent assistants and two other people with a handicap. Claudia was able to receive the attention she needed from Nadine, who was responsible for the house and had a very close relationship with her. Claudia spent a lot of time with Nadine, who knew how to touch and bathe her and how to speak to her in a warm, comforting tone of voice. She also knew how to be firm when necessary.

Gradually Claudia became less frightened and insecure. She began to realise that somebody loved her and valued her and that she must therefore be lovable. The regular routine (bath, meal, school, prayers, playtime) and the loving care she received from Nadine and the others helped her greatly. But it was a long process, taking several years, and the community needed help and advice from a good psychiatrist, who helped the assistants to understand what was happening to Claudia and how to respond. He also prescribed medication to calm her and help her to sleep.

Claudia has changed a great deal. She will always be blind and 'autistic' and relationships are still difficult, but she has found an inner peace and her face is much less anguished. She is a young woman with a secure home and people to turn to. She has even started to sing to herself.

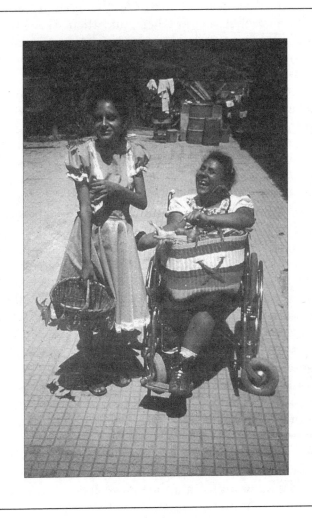

Claudia and Marcia from l'Arche Honduras

Compassion is not the suppression of suffering, but the willingness to bear it alongside the grieving person. When a mother has lost her child there is no way of dispelling her grief, but we can be there, weeping and praying with her. She needs to know that she is not alone but has a loving friend to support and encourage her.

Compassion is presence, a way of enabling the grief-stricken person to know that someone is with them and that there is a way forward. During his agony Jesus showed his need of the three apostles, – 'Could you not watch one hour with me?' and he suffered even more because they fell asleep.

A person in deep distress is in danger of falling into despair which is a taste of death. A compassionate friend will help that person to go through the grief and mourning, bringing a tiny flicker of hope which comes from the heart of God and gives a meaning to their suffering. We discover then that through all the pain we are participating in the Cross of Jesus for the salvation of the world. This is perhaps the most difficult, even the most impossible, aspect of compassion and the reason that it is essentially a gift of God. In the presence of another person's grief I tend to try and 'do' something in order to assuage my own anguish. But to remain present to that person, while doing nothing, but with a heart filled with hope, like Mary at the foot of the Cross, demands a special gift of the Holy Spirit.

We cannot be compassionate unless we are aware of our own shortcomings – our poverty. We cannot enter into the suffering of another if we have not accepted our own suffering and the fact that we too are on the road to death. This is the reality of our common creatureliness and dependence. Only when we discover that God forgives our sin and rebellion can we begin to forgive the sin and rebellion of others. If we remain unaware of our sinfulness and therefore unaware of the mercy of God, we are in danger of going to the poor as a 'have' doing good to the 'have nots'. The recipient of our 'generosity' may be grateful for any help and advice, but will not feel that he or she has been deeply understood. We cannot approach the suffering of others unless we have suffered ourselves.

I lived some deep experiences in a Haitian prison. These men and women were violent, primitive and deeply frustrated; in the front row were twenty women, in the second twenty men, and behind them in a wooden cage were some hundred other men. I was put at the front to talk and at first all the faces were closed up. I felt that I was being rejected because I was a white man from outside and they were expecting some sort of a sermon.

I started to talk about children – the child within each one of them and within me. I spoke of the child's yearning for tenderness; of the way these men and women saw themselves and the way I saw myself. At the end I said, 'Maybe some of you will never get out of this prison, or will only get out in order to be brought back a few weeks later. You may be rejected by everybody, but I hope that one day the world will discover the beauty within you. My hope is that one day we will live a resurrection and that your inner beauty will then burst forth and be recognised by all. You know, as I know, that deep within you, beyond everything that has gone wrong, there is a child yearning for tenderness.'

Faces relaxed, began to smile, there was a moment of communion between us, a moment of peace. Maybe for some that moment of peace will flow into their consciousness at the time of their death and make it possible for them to trust.

At l'Arche our basic philosophy is that of learning to be happy together.

We believe that the joy of friendship comes before independence. Joy says, 'I am happy that you exist,' and thus transforms the broken self-image of the other person. Any form of training which gives primacy to autonomy without this basis of joy in togetherness can be seen as a sort of rejection: 'I want you to be self-sufficient so that I won't have to live with you.' It can force the other person to prove themselves in a way that does not help them to grow interiorly.

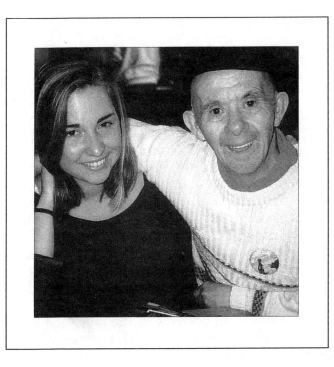

Sarah and Bertie at l'Arche Edinburgh

It is wonderful to see how the Catholic Church has kept its sense of celebration. Almost every day is a feast-day – either a great liturgical festival or a saint's day. And then at the heart of each day we celebrate the Eucharist. I am always struck by the vocabulary of the Eucharist: celebration and feast, presence and communion, meal and sacrifice, forgiveness and thanksgiving.

Celebration is a cry of joy and gratitude that our lives are bound together, linked one to another in trust as part of a single body in which difference is seen as a treasure. Barriers that separate us from one another can disappear and we rejoice as we reveal to one another what is deepest and most vulnerable in us.

Celebration is an overflow of the unity and sense of communion between members of a community. It is the peak of community life, a means of creating and expressing unity.

And every human reality has a part in the celebration: mind and body, music and dancing, food and fun, happiness and laughter, flowers, beautiful things, our best clothes.

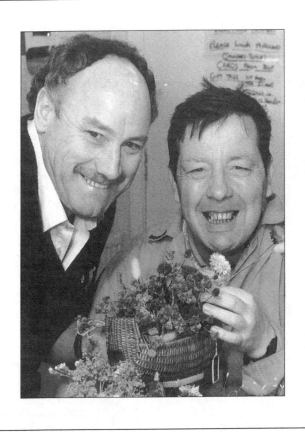

Brian and Derek at Inverness

At the heart of celebration, there are the poor. If the least significant is excluded, it is no longer a celebration. We have to find dances and games in which the children, the old people and the weak can join equally. A celebration must always be a festival of the poor, and with the poor, not for the poor.

And celebration is the sign that beyond all the sufferings, purifications and deaths, there is the eternal wedding feast, the great celebration of life with God. It is the sign that there is a personal meeting which will fulfil us, that our thirst for the infinite will be slaked and that the wound of our loneliness will be healed.

Fifteen of Pierre's twenty years have been spent in the psychiatric hospital where he was placed at the age of two. Pierre understands very little but suffers a lot, although he finds it hard to communicate because his sight and hearing are limited.

The other evening he had a high temperature, and while I was sitting beside his bed he gave a little smile and stretched out to take my hand. We stayed like that, hand in hand, happy just to be together, and I found that I was praying. Pierre's trust touched me very deeply: our clasped hands a sign of the covenant between us.

WALK HUMBLY
WITH YOUR GOD

The poor
are not there just to receive our charity:
they are sources of life and truth,
peacemakers.
This, then, is the great secret of Jesus,
hidden in the Gospels.

Many people see them
as a sign of death, source of despair;
a problem, a burden,
people to be pushed aside, perhaps eliminated,
forced to change their ways.

Jesus shows us
that the poor can transform our hearts,
filling us with light and compassion,
if we are willing to accept to meet them
and live in communion with them.

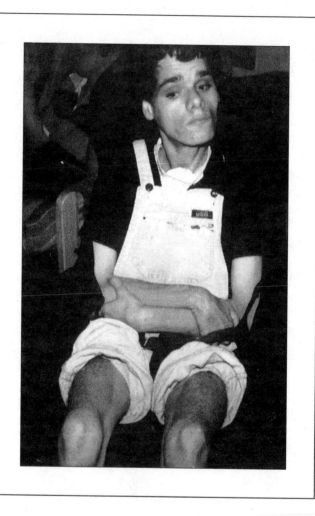

Eric at Trosly-Breuil

Eric has taught me so much. He has taught me that the Father, if he is hidden in the beauties of creation and in the grandeur of worship and in the wisdom of theologians and scientists, is also hidden in the broken bodies of the lepers, the sick and the suffering. He is hidden in the child.

> Whosoever welcomes one of these little ones in My name, welcomes Me. And whosoever welcomes Me, says Jesus, welcomes the One who sent Me. (Luke 9: 48)

Who can believe in this message: that the Eternal and Almighty God is to be found in the little ones, in the powerless, in the crushed and suffering ones of the world, and that to live with them is to live with the Divine Trinity – Father, Son and Spirit? As Jesus is icon of the Father, so is the abandoned, rejected child icon of Jesus, and as we enter into a relationship of trust with him, we enter into a relationship of trust with God.

> Surely he has borne our griefs and carried our sorrows; with his stripes we are healed. (Isa. 53: 4–5)

Eric has revealed to me that what is most precious in me is my heart. He has shown me that my head and hands are of value only to the degree that they are at the service of love and covenant relationships that flow from the covenant with Jesus. His weakness, his fragility, his trust, have awakened me and called me forth, and, I dare say, are leading me on the road to healing and wholeness. He is calling me from the isolation of my pride, and of my fears, into compassion, understanding, tenderness and community.

The poor are prophetic. They call us to change and to discover a new way of life: a real encounter with one another in celebration and forgiveness. But we often shut ourselves away in our wealth and isolation, rushing from one pastime to another. We are frightened of the poor who invite us to experience real tenderness and deep communion. We have no idea how to respond to such an invitation and although we may be well educated and intelligent, able to do all sorts of things, our hearts are underdeveloped – possibly because we are frightened. The relationship into which we are called is not one of sentimentality or fleeting emotion: still less is it a romantic encounter or a sexual experience. Rather, it is an invitation to deep trust and the mutual recognition of gifts.

We are in danger of self-sufficiency, shut away in the prison of our power and security. The poor can turn all that upside down, breaking down the barriers and allowing a sort of miracle to take place if we will only allow it to happen. A deep encounter with the poor brings new life and a real meeting in which it is possible to discover that we too have hearts to love – and at the same time we become aware of our fears and barriers: the search for comfort and security.

If, once our hearts are touched, we allow ourselves to respond to the poor, we may gradually discover a power and hidden energy welling up from a deeper source than our knowledge and our capacity for 'doing'. We may also find an unsuspected ability to meet and serve others, thus becoming a sign of the love of God. We will find the strength of tenderness, goodness, patience, forgiveness, joy and celebration: a sealed spring bursting forth.

The broken Body of the Church
is the source of so many tears.

Maybe today Christians are not fully one
in their beliefs, their organisation and their struc-
tures.
But they can be one in their love
and in their yearning to follow Jesus,
not always knowing the path ahead,
which will be revealed little by little by the Spirit.

They can be one
as together they walk down the ladder with Jesus,
meeting Jesus in the poorest and the weakest.

It is true
that Christians cannot all eat today around the same
    table
of the broken bread,
transformed into the Body of Christ,
but they can eat together
around the same table
with the poor and the weak.

Is not this the most direct path to unity?

Moments of communion with the poor can become times of prayer and union with Jesus, who himself becomes the link between us. This, surely, is the meaning of his new commandment: to love one another with his love. There is a stillness, a presence of God in the loving, welcoming gestures of the poor: in their tenderness and steadfastness. If I am to discover that the poor are an outward sign of inward grace – a sacrament – I must try to live in the presence of Jesus. Real communion can spring up between us – deep meeting which is a gift of God – gift, one to another. Our way of caring must be deeply sensitive, filled with gentleness, peace, openness. We are bound together in mutual tenderness and trust – an experience of grace.

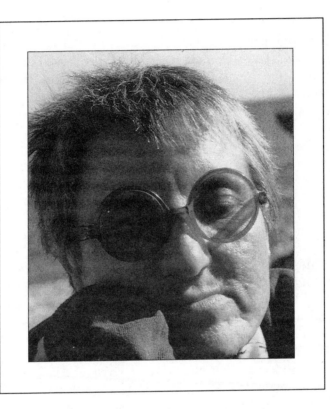

Janet from l' Arche Bognor Regis

Walking with the poor, I have touched on my own poverty. Their wounds have revealed mine. They have shown me my fears of truly following Jesus in trust, humility and poverty, and how often I wanted to flee, to hide in knowledge, in dreams for tomorrow, in power, or in human security.

Yes, the poor disturb me. Their prophetic cry for understanding, friendship and opportunity, has revealed to me my hardness, selfishness, sin and my resistance to change. They have revealed how imprisoned I am in my own fears and in my own culture.

And yet I know that my covenant is with them, that in them and with them I meet Jesus Christ; Jesus, hidden in the hungry, the thirsty, the homeless, the naked, the stranger, the sick, the prisoner: Jesus, Life of the world. And I must learn to meet Jesus not only in the poverty of Paul, but also in my own poverty. I need Jesus, our Saviour, to teach me to love. Yes, I know it is true: Jesus the Lover is hidden in the wounds of Paul, Eric, Claudia and Innocente, but also in my own wounds.

His wounded and pierced heart is hidden in the littleness and weakness and wounds of humanity.

We are called not only to work with all our might for a better world and to relieve suffering wherever we find it, but to enter into ever deeper communion with those who suffer, respecting them in their weakness and frailty, and still more in the mystery of their suffering.

There is a secret meaning and beauty in the lives of these sick, feeble, rejected, 'useless' people which is vital. Far from being 'failures' or 'useless', they are the invisible underground roots beneath the great tree of humanity: that abandoned child, this man in trouble with the police, the mother with a son who drinks too much, that girl with a mental handicap, old people, prisoners, the dying.

We see trunk, branches, leaves and fruit – we respect the strong, clever and powerful – those with outstanding achievements to their name – and we ignore the roots: poor, feeble, disadvantaged men and women, hidden in the darkness, giving life to the tree.

It is not their suffering which is the source of life, but he who by his love chose to share our human suffering, transforming it into a sign of his presence among us: a sacrament.

So, do not shrink from suffering,
but enter into it
and discover there the mystery
of the presence of the risen Jesus.
He is hidden there, in the sacrament of the poor.

And do not turn aside from your own pain,
your anguish and brokenness,
your loneliness and emptiness,
by pretending you are strong.

Go within yourself.
Go down the ladder of your own being
until you discover –
like a seed
buried in the broken, ploughed earth
of your own vulnerability –
the presence of Jesus,
the light shining in the darkness.

And there, offer yourself with Jesus
to the Father
for the life of the world.

Today as yesterday
Jesus is calling us to follow him,
to walk in his footsteps.

He is calling you and me to be like him,
wherever and whoever we are,
whatever we think of ourselves.

To live as he lived,
to love as he loved,
to speak as he spoke,
to offer our lives as he offered his,
to do what he did,
to do even greater things
because of his going to the Father.

The good news is that God so loves us all and came to bring us freedom. This freedom comes through the love and tenderness of Jesus as he reveals himself to us and helps us to understand his message.

'I am with you, holding you close in all your poverty and weakness. You do not have to be afraid because I am always with you. I have not come to condemn you but to forgive, so there is no need to be frightened of your weakness and egoism.

'Be yourself without anxiety because I understand you and I have come to take from your flesh the heart of stone and to teach you to love.'

In order that his divine presence and the power of the Spirit may enter into us, Jesus asks only one thing: that we become like the poor, opening our hearts to him, believing in his power to heal.

Jesus says, 'Dare to love, dare to hold out your hand to another person. Perhaps you will do stupid things, but it doesn't matter. You are the channel for my faithfulness so do not be afraid of your infidelity.'

It is important to realise that, left to ourselves, we cannot be faithful. There is no such thing as true, life-giving love unless it comes from the heart of Jesus. Love is always possessive unless it is grounded in God – we take and possess, and seek to be admired by others, rather than to give life.

It is impossible to be close to a wounded person, respecting his or her fears and accepting minimal progress, unless we are close to Jesus and the Holy Spirit. They alone can give the inner peace and strength which we need in order to love in a way that enables the person with a handicap to realise that he or she too is lifegiving: a love that is not self-serving, manipulative or in search of personal prestige.

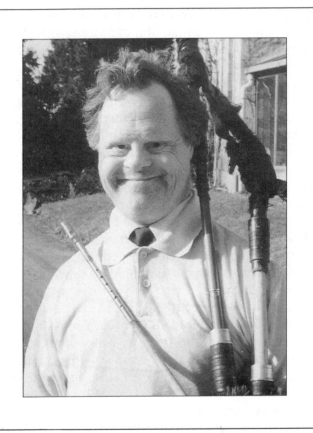

Cathol from Inverness

During the moments of communion with Eric, as well as during more difficult moments with him, I discovered more than ever before that forgiveness is at the heart of l'Arche. It is at the heart of any relationship simply because we are men and women wounded in our hearts and our affectivity. We have built up a whole system of defence and aggression around our vulnerability.

When Eric closes up in himself, when he cuts himself off from relationship, he needs to feel that his anger and refusal are forgiven. He must not feel condemned or judged. Anger or aggression must not signify breaking off a relationship. No, it is only a temporary breakage which can be repaired. Refusal and aggression can, through reconciliation, be transformed into communion. Eric needs to sense that he has been forgiven, just as I need to feel I have been forgiven. For I, too, need reconciliation.

The celebration of forgiveness is a deep liberation which is communicated from one person to another: 'you are aggressive, enclosed; perhaps there is much hatred and fear in you; but hidden beneath all that, there is your heart. There is your deepest self where God dwells and there, I love you.'

When I hear those words or when I sense them, it is my deepest self, the heart of my heart, that is revealed to me. If someone can see light in a corner of my being, then there is hope. And hope is the birth, the rebirth of vital energy.

In order to penetrate this world of forgiveness, we must experience the forgiveness of God that is given to us by Jesus. The mystery Jesus came to reveal to us is just that: that God does not condemn or judge us. He comes to break down the barriers of hatred and to help us enter into the celebration of reconciliation.

If we want to grow in love we have to be patient and not expect to 'see' things, any more than we can expect to see a plant in the act of growing.

It is the same with the life of grace – we have to allow the Holy Spirit to fill us slowly and gently with his life and peace.

It can be difficult to know when the Spirit is at work in me and frequently I can only tell by results – the peace he puts into my heart.

But the Holy Spirit is a gift of God which is called to bear fruit – not just a sense of peace, but an enfolding of body and soul so that I start to love God with all my heart and with every fibre of my being. I must be completely transformed by the Holy Spirit so as to radiate the Beatitudes and bring peace and reconciliation to a world of hatred, division and exploitation.

Prayer is entering gently and peacefully into the silence of Jesus, allowing him to give himself to me; my heart beating at the rhythm of his heart, my breathing in tune with his. As I become increasingly aware of God within, I enter ever more deeply into this presence; not so as to flee from my brothers and sisters but in order to become more present to them. It is impossible to approach the crucified Christ without coming closer to all those who are crucified today.

When my prayer becomes a cry from the depths of my being, imploring God to send his peace and remove my fears and barriers, it is the Holy Spirit who comes, bringing new hope and breaking down the walls. The Spirit enters into my life in a way that is appropriate to my age, circumstances and spiritual development. When God seems to have vanished, Emmanuel – the God with us – is still present and often seems furthest when closest. The night is darkest just before the dawn.

81

A Door of Hope

The Vale of Achor is the valley of misfortune
a dangerous valley close to Jericho
an accursed place
swarming with insects and poisonous creatures
a place to flee
a place of pain
a place of your pain
a place to avoid
to dread
to keep out of
to try to forget
a place of the poor, suffering, desperate and disinherited
those you avoid
reject, hide
try to forget about
And yet God says:
'I will make the Vale of Achor
a door of hope' (Hosea 2:15)
That is the mystery: God says
if you do not run away
if you dare to enter the place of pain
within your own heart
if you welcome
those you fear
those you reject
those who threaten you
because they are poor and weak and wounded
among them the wounded child within you:
the child who you shut away
behind a high wall
long ago:
if you welcome that child
and welcome yourself
you will be on the road to healing
and the Vale of Achor
will become a door of Hope.

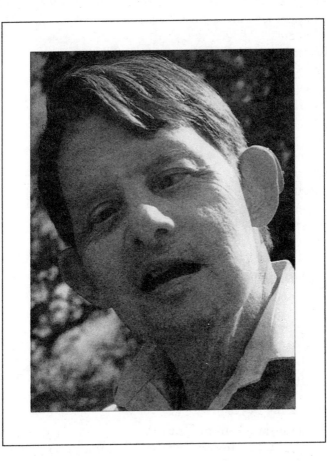

Nick at l'Arche Lambeth

Sources

Introduction

Following Jesus

Act Justly

was first published by Pastorale-Quebec in the same year and reproduced with their permission as *Une Esperance* (Les Chemins de L'Arche-La-Ferme) from which this translation was made (p 8).

35 Slightly adapted from *Tears of Silence*, p 34.

36 Translated from 'L'Acceuil . . . ça dérange' in *Ombres et Lumières*, no. 70, June 1985, pp 26, 27.

37 Slightly adapted from Jean Vanier, *Be Not Afraid*, 1993 (Dublin: Gill & Macmillan), p 117.

39 Jean Vanier, *Our Inner Journey* (Richmond Hill, Ontario: Daybreak), pp 30, 31, 32.

41 *Our Inner Journey*, pp 38–9.

42 First two paragraphs: translation, unidentified source. Third paragraph: slightly adapted from Jean Vanier, *Community and Growth*, revised edition, 1989 (London: Darton, Longman & Todd), p 264.

44 *Our Inner Journey*, pp 33–4.

Love Tenderly

47 *The Broken Body*, pp 19–20.

49 Translation: unidentified source.

50 Translation: unidentified source.

52 Translation: unidentified source.

53 Slightly adapted from *Eruption to Hope*, pp 11, 12.

54 *Tears of Silence*, pp 76, 78.

55 *The Broken Body*, pp 52, 53.

56 Translated from Jean Vanier, *Communauté et Croissance* (Les Chemins de l'Arche-La-Ferme), pp 3–4.

58 From an article in *Christus*, no. 111, June 1981. Reproduced as *Au Coeur de la Compassion* (Les Chemins de l'Arche-La-Ferme), from which this translation was made.

59 Translated from *La Peur d'Aimer*, pp 11–13.

60 Translated from *Solidaire de Tous* (Les Chemins de

l'Arche-La-Ferme), the transcription of an interview with Rémi Montour, p 6.

62 First paragraph from *Community and Growth*, p 321. Remainder of the page translated from an unidentified source.

64 First two paragraphs from *Community and Growth*, pp 319, 331. Last two paragraphs translated from *Au Coeur de la Compassion*, pp 11–12.

Walk Humbly With Your God

67 Translation: unidentified source.

69 From the keynote address to the World Council of Churches meeting in Vancouver, British Columbia, in 1983, published as *The Poor, a Path to Unity* (Les Chemins de l'Arche-La-Ferme), from which this extract is slightly adapted (pp 6, 8).

70 Adapted from *To Welcome the Poor is to Welcome Jesus* (Les Chemins de l'Arche-La-Ferme), p 10.

71 *The Broken Body*, pp 132–3.

72 Translation: unidentified source.

74 Slightly adapted from Jean Vanier, *The Poor, a Path to Unity* (Les Chemins de l'Arche-La-Ferme), p 9.

75 Translation: unidentified source.

76 Slightly adapted from *The Broken Body*, pp 62–3.

77 *The Broken Body*, pp 68–9.

78 Translation: unidentified source.

80 *Our Inner Journey*, pp 12, 13.

81 Translation: unidentified source.

82 Translation: written by Jean Vanier for the French edition of this book.

List of English Texts
by Jean Vanier Used in This Book

Books

Be Not Afraid, 1993 [1976] (Dublin: Gill & Macmillan).
The Broken Body, 1988 (London: Darton, Longman & Todd).
Community and Growth, revised edition, 1989 (London: Darton, Longman & Todd).
Eruption to Hope, 1971 (Toronto: Griffin Press).
Man and Woman He Made Them, 1985 (London: Darton, Longman & Todd).
Tears of Silence, 1970 (London: Darton, Longman & Todd).

Pamphlets

Our Inner Journey (Richmond Hill, Ontario: Daybreak).
The Poor, a Path to Unity (Trosly–Breuil, France: Les Chemins de l'Arche–La–Ferme).
To Welcome the Poor is to Welcome Jesus (Trosly–Breuil, France: Les Chemins de l'Arche–La–Ferme).

Related titles

Jean Vanier and l'Arche: a Communion of Love, Kathryn Spink, 1990 (London: Dalton, Longman & Todd).

The Road to Daybreak, Henri J.M. Nouwen, 1988 (London: Dalton, Longman & Todd).
Nick: Man of the Heart, Thérèse Vanier, 1993 (Dublin: Gill & Macmillan).
Treasures of the Heart: Daily Readings with Jean Vanier, ed. Sister Benedict, 1989 (London: Darton Longman & Todd).

Whereas a single publisher is given for each of the books listed above, a number of them are available through publishing houses in other English-speaking countries.

Details of publications as well as information on other documentation and audio-visual material is available as follows:

UK: L'Arche Secretariat
10 Briggate
Silsden
Keighley
West Yorkshire BD20 9JT

Canada and USA:
Daybreak Publications
11339 Yonge Street
Richmond Hill
Ontario L4C 4X7

Further Information

For further information on **l'Arche** communities in English-speaking countries:

Australia:
L'Arche–Genesaret
PO Box 734
Woden
ACT 2606

Canada:
Daybreak
11339 Yonge Street
Richmond Hill
Ontario
L4C 4X7

Ireland:
L'Arche Cork
102 Elm Park
Wilton
Cork

UK:
L'Arche Secretariat
10 Briggate
Silsden
Keighley
West Yorkshire BD20 9JT

United States:
L'Arche–Erie
523 West 8th Street
Erie
Pa 16502

For further information on **Faith and Light** communities in English-speaking countries:

Australia/Asia:
Lucina Bourke
51 Allawah
Blacktown
NSW 2148
Australia

Ireland:
Hannah O'Brien
Inchnagree
Buttevant
Cork

UK:
Cecilia Horsburgh
Cranham
3 Forestfield
Kelso
Roxburghshire TD5 7BX

USA:
Mr and Mrs Dani
2354 E. Briarhurst Drive
Highlands Ranch
CO 80126

Faith and Light International Secretariat
3 rue de Laos
75105 Paris
France